Simply Svelte: 30 Days to Thin

SIMPLY SVELTE

HEALTHY EATING MADE EASY

ISBN-13: 978-0988354746

FIRST THINGS FIRST

Consult with your physician before beginning any diet and/or exercise program.

CONTENTS

1	What Weight Makes You Feel Great?	1
2	30 Days to Thin	3
3	How to Follow the Plan	5
4	Mix-and-Match 300-Calorie Meals	7
	About Simply Svelte	48

1
WHAT WEIGHT MAKES YOU FEEL GREAT?

Chances are, at some point in the past, you've weighed what you would consider your ideal weight. Maybe it was a LONG time ago. Maybe you were even a teenager. Even if it's been years since you felt confident with your weight, stop for a moment and try to remember what it felt like.

You know you're at a healthy weight when:

- The clothes in your closet fit well and flatter you.
- You feel energetic and ready to conquer your day.
- Your family and friends tell you how great you look.
- You feel sexy.
- You glow.

What is that weight? Stop for a moment and think of a number—a reasonable number based on your height. If you need help understanding what constitutes a healthy weight for your height, use one of the many online calculators that will give you a range from low to high.

Once you know your ideal weight—that number that allows you to put on anything in your closet and feel great—write it down. If you're a woman, multiply by 13. If you're a man, multiply by 17.

The result is how many calories you need to eat consistently, EVERY SINGLE DAY in order to reach and maintain that ideal number you have in mind.

Example:
If you are a woman who wants to weigh 120 pounds:

120 pounds x 13 = 1,560 calories

You would need to eat 1,560 calories consistently—every day—in order to reach your ideal weight.

Your body is amazingly adaptable. It will adjust to whatever you do on a regular basis. That's why habits are so important! If you eat the same number of calories each day, your body will adapt. It will naturally begin to shed pounds to adjust to your new daily caloric intake.

Once you know the number of calories you need to eat each day to reach your ideal weight, then it must be time to start counting calories. But wait! If you've ever tried to count calories before, you know how tedious and time-consuming it can be. You might feel ready to give up even before you get started.

That's where the Simply Svelte 30 Days to Thin comes in. We've broken down breakfast, lunch, dinner and snacks into easy 300-calorie chunks. All you do is mix and match these 300-calorie units to add up to your daily calorie allotment. If your daily calorie allotment falls slightly above or below the 1500, 1800, or 2100-calorie mark, just shave off a few bites or add a few more.

We've tried to make this program as easy as possible to follow, and to make sure that every bite you put into your mouth is nutritious and delicious.

For the next 30 days, give it a fair trial. We think you'll be amazed how you look and feel one month from today.

2
30 DAYS TO THIN

The Simply Svelte 30 Days to Thin is founded on four simple, sensible food staples:

- Olive oil: Use it sparingly, as it packs 120 calories per tablespoon. Choose it over butter and any other kind of oil. Olive oil is healthy, all-natural, and has a wonderful flavor. To minimize the calories, use olive oil cooking spray in some recipes.

- Fresh fruits and vegetables: Aim to make at least half of your diet consist of fruits and vegetables. The more raw fruits and vegetables you eat, the better your level of overall nutrition.

- Lean meats: Limit consumption of red meat to no more than once per week. Stock up on fish, poultry, and lean cuts of pork, lamb, and beef.

- Whole grains: The fewer you eat, the faster the pounds will drop.

However, don't eliminate grains entirely or the pounds will pack back on quickly as soon as you reintroduce them. Aim for one to two meals with whole grains each day—brown rice, whole-wheat pasta and 100% whole-grain bread.

You decide how much to eat. You choose the daily caloric intake that will allow you to lose weight and feel satisfied. Is it 1200 calories? 1500? 1800? 2100? You decide. Simply mix and match 300-calorie options to customize a menu that's right for you. For example, a typical 1,500-calorie day might looks like this:

- 8:00am: Breakfast
- 10:30am: Mid-morning snack
- 1:00pm: Lunch
- 3:30pm: Mid-afternoon snack
- 6:30pm: Dinner

Read on for delicious breakfasts, lunches, dinners, and snacks. Each one equals approximately 300 calories. Every day, mix and match to choose a combination that's right for you! These are some of the easiest recipes on earth to make.

You don't have to be an accomplished chef to prepare delicious, nutritious recipes that you and your family will love. Best of all, they'll help you establish the daily habits that will take off the pounds—and keep them off.

3
HOW TO FOLLOW THE PLAN

Step 1: Clean out your pantry.

Start by stripping your kitchen of anything that will tempt you to overeat. Common "trigger foods" include potato chips, cookies, snack crackers, and ice cream, but it's different for everyone. You know what your own trigger foods are. Get rid of them!

In addition, some things in your kitchen are just plain bad for you. In the interest of improving your overall health—and losing weight—you'll want to banish these items from your pantry for good:

- Sodas, regular or diet
- Anything with hydrogenated oils and/or corn syrup
- Refined carbohydrates (white bread and pasta, for example)
- Most packaged foods (cookies, snack crackers, junk food)

Step 2: Go shopping.

Now that you've cleaned out your pantry, it's time to fill it back up—with the right stuff! Each week, buy fresh produce and meat. Make sure that the following items are stocked in your kitchen at all times:

Pantry Staples:

- Extra-virgin olive oil
- Balsamic vinegar
- Boxed chicken and vegetable broth (organic if possible)
- Olive oil cooking spray

- Canned or dried beans (chick peas, kidney beans)
- Whole wheat pasta
- Brown rice

Refrigerator Staples:

- Cooked rotisserie chicken (organic if possible)
- Lean, spiral sliced ham
- Lean deli turkey
- Fat-free cheddar and/or feta cheese
- Skim (fat-free) milk

Freezer Staples:

- Frozen fruit for smoothies
- Frozen mixed vegetables (organic if possible)
- Frozen individual portions of salmon steaks, cooked shrimp

Step 3: Mix and match your meals.
Mix and match the 300-calorie breakfasts, lunches, dinners and snacks contained in this book. If you want to eat a 1,500-calorie menu, choose a breakfast, lunch, dinner, and two snacks. Choosing 1,800 calories might earn you breakfast, lunch, dinner, plus three snacks. You decide, based on your own body's needs.

Step 4: Track your meals, watch your drinks.
Keep track of your meals and snacks. Research has shown that people who write down what they eat are more successful at losing weight and keeping it off. Limit drinks to water, tea, and black coffee. Ditch the soft drinks. Sodas—even diet ones—are not only full of unhealthy chemicals, but they've been proven to sabotage your diet. Start eating clean, and those diet sodas you were once addicted to will start to taste artificial and disgusting!

Step 5: Track your weight loss.
When you weigh yourself every day, you'll learn quickly what works for you. You'll also learn that your weight may fluctuate with normal hormonal changes each month, and you'll understand exactly what impact a candy bar can have! Track your progress day by day, and check it each week to see how you're doing overall.

Step 6: Enjoy the results!
Don't forget to congratulate yourself on a job well done!

4
MIX-AND-MATCH 300-CALORIE MEALS

BREAKFAST

*Breakfast recipes denoted with an asterisk (*) can be found in 300-Calorie Breakfast: 30 Days of Healthy, Hassle-Free Recipes from the editors of Simply Svelte.

ALMOND BUTTER SANDWICH | GRAPEFRUIT

2 slices light 100% whole wheat bread (140 calories)
1 Tbsp almond butter (101 calories)
1 whole medium grapefruit (41 calories)

Total calories = 282

ALMOND BUTTER STRAWBERRY & HONEY SANDWICH

2 slices sprouted grain bread (160 calories)
1 Tbsp almond butter (101 calories)
1 tsp honey (35 calories)
5 strawberries, sliced thinly (19 calories)

Total calories = 315

Asparagus Frittata | Toast | Yogurt | Strawberries

*Asparagus Frittata (78 calories)
1 slice 100% whole grain bread, toasted (100 calories)
1 cup sliced strawberries (53 calories)
1 cup fat-free Greek yogurt (60 calories)

Total calories = 291

Banana Almond Oatmeal

1 cup oatmeal cooked in water (129 calories)
1 medium banana, sliced (53 calories)
15 whole almonds (104 calories)

Total calories = 286

Bagel with Cream Cheese | Blueberries

1 whole wheat "mini bagel" or 1 regular whole wheat bagel (150 calories)
1 oz light cream cheese (70 calories)
1 cup blueberries (83 calories)

Total calories = 286

BLUEBERRY PANCAKES

2 pancakes made from 100% whole grain mix (184 calories)
1 Tbsp pure natural maple syrup (52 calories)
1 cup fresh blueberries (63 calories)

Total calories = 299

BREAKFAST BURRITO

1 whole wheat tortilla (120 calories)
1/4 cup black beans, drained (55 calories)
1 cup tomato salsa (17 calories)
2 scrambled egg whites (34 calories)
1 oz fat-free cheddar cheese, shredded (42 calories)
2 oz fat-free sour cream (42 calories)

Total calories = 310

BREAKFAST SMOOTHIE

1 cup fat-free plain yogurt
2 oz skim (fat-free) milk
1 cup frozen mixed berries
1 Tbsp honey

Total calories = 285

Canadian Bacon & Eggs | Grits | Orange

1 slice Canadian Bacon served with 2 scrambled egg whites and 1 oz fat-free cheddar cheese (164 calories)
1 cup instant grits, cooked (107 calories)
1 small orange (45 calories)

Total calories = 291

Cereal | Raspberries

2 ounces whole-grain cereal (Grape Nuts, Total, puffed brown rice) (200 calories)
1 cup skim milk (45 calories)
1 cup raspberries (32 calories)

Total calories = 277

Cereal | Hard-Boiled Egg

2 ounces whole-grain cereal (Grape Nuts, Total, puffed brown rice) (200 calories)
1 cup skim milk (45 calories)
1 hardboiled egg (78 calories)

Total calories = 323

Cereal | Yogurt | Banana

2 ounces whole-grain cereal (Grape Nuts, Total, puffed brown rice) (200 calories)
1 container fat-free, fruit-flavored yogurt (50 calories)
1 medium banana (53 calories)

Total calories = 303

Cheese Grits Casserole | Strawberries

*Cheese Grits Casserole, 1-cup serving (280 calories)
1 cup sliced strawberries (27 calories)

Total calories = 295

Cheese Omelet | Toast | Blueberries

Cheese Omelet made with 2 egg whites and 1 oz fat-free cheddar cheese (76 calories)
1 slice 100% whole grain bread, toasted (100 calories)
1 cup blueberries (83 calories)

Total calories = 259

Cheesy Toast | Raspberries

2 slices 100% whole grain bread (200 calories)
2 oz non-fat cheddar cheese, melted on bread under the broiler (84)
1 cup raspberries (32)

Total calories = 316

Chinese Breakfast | Apple

*Chinese Breakfast (230 calories)
1 small apple (77 calories)

Total calories = 307

English Muffin Breakfast Sandwich | Orange

1 whole wheat English muffin (120 calories)
2 scrambled egg whites (34 calories)
1 oz fat-free cheddar cheese, shredded (42 calories)
1 small orange (45 calories)

Total calories = 285

FRESH HERB FRITTATA | TOAST | PEAR

*Fresh Herb Frittata (151 calories)
1 slice 100% whole grain bread, toasted (100 calories)
½ cup blueberries (42 calories)

Total calories = 293

GREEK OMELET | CANADIAN BACON | GRITS | ORANGE

*Greek Omelet (87 calories)
1 serving (3/4 cup cooked) instant grits (107 calories)
1 slice Canadian bacon (44 calories)
1 small orange (45 calories)

Total calories = 283

HOME FRIES | STRAWBERRIES

*Home Fries (288 calories)
1 cup sliced strawberries (53 calories)

Total calories = 341

Hot and Spicy Eggs | Toast | Banana

*Hot and Spicy Eggs (222 calories)
1 medium banana (105 calories)

Total calories = 327

Italian Wrap | Banana

Italian Wrap (235 calories)
1 cup sliced strawberries (53 calories)

Total calories = 288

Mushroom Scramble | Polenta | Canadian Bacon

*Mushroom Scramble (165 calories)
1 cup polenta, cooked (126 calories)

Total calories = 291

Peanut Butter Banana | Cheerios

1 medium banana, sliced lengthwise (106 calories)
1 Tbsp organic peanut butter (105 calories)
1 cup multigrain Cheerios (55 calories)
1 cup skim milk (45 calories)

Total calories = 311

Peanut Butter Breakfast Sandwich

2 slices light whole wheat bread (140 calories)
1 Tbsp organic peanut butter (105 calories)
1 medium banana, sliced and layered on sandwich (53 calories)

Total calories = 298

Poached Egg with Tomato | Ham | Raspberries

*Poached Egg with Tomato (243 calories)
1 cup raspberries (32 calories)

Total calories = 275

South-of-the-Border Eggs | Orange

*South-of-the-Border Eggs (244 calories)
1 small orange (45 calories)

Total calories = 289

Spinach Feta Omelet | Toast | Banana

*Spinach Feta Omelet (79 calories)
1 slice 100% whole grain bread, toasted (100 calories)
1 medium banana (105 calories)

Total calories = 280

Steak, Pepper and Egg Souffle | Strawberries

*Steak, Pepper, and Egg Souffle (264 calories)
1 cup sliced fresh strawberries (53 calories)

Total calories = 317

STRAWBERRY FLAXSEED OATMEAL WITH ALMONDS

1 cup oatmeal cooked in water (129 calories)
1 cup sliced strawberries (27 calories)
1 Tbsp flaxseed (40 calories)
1 cup slivered almonds (133 calories)

Total calories = 329

LUNCH

*Lunch recipes denoted with an asterisk (*) can be found in 300-Calorie Lunch: 30 Days of Healthy, Hassle-Free Recipes from the editors of Simply Svelte.

BBQ PULLED PORK SANDWICH | ORANGE BELL PEPPER

*BBQ Pulled Pork Sandwich (308 calories)
1 cup orange bell pepper, cut into strips (18 calories)

Total calories = 326

BLACK BEAN QUESADILLA

*Black Bean Quesadilla (334 calories)

Total calories = 334

BREADLESS BLT | BLACK BEAN SOUP | TANGERINE

1 slice of Canadian bacon, 2 slices tomato, and 1 tsp fat-free mayonnaise, wrapped in 2 Romaine lettuce leaves (130 calories)
1 cup black bean soup, canned (130 calories)
1 small tangerine (40 calories)

Total calories = 300

CARROT SOUP | TOAST WITH HUMMUS | STRAWBERRIES

*2 cups Carrot Soup (160 calories)
1 slice 100% whole grain bread, toasted (100 calories)
1 Tablespoon hummus (23 calories)
1 cup sliced strawberries (27 calories)

Total calories = 310

CHICKEN AND BROWN RICE SALAD

*Chicken and Brown Rice Salad (308 calories)

Total calories = 308

Chicken Burrito to Go

*Chicken Burrito to Go (305 calories)

Total calories = 305

Chicken Noodle Soup

*Chicken Noodle Soup (292 calories)

Total calories = 292

Chicken Salad Pita

*Chicken Salad Pita (329 calories)

Total calories = 329

Hearty Bean Salad

*Hearty Bean Salad (301 calories)

Total calories = 301

Lentil Salad | Baby Carrots

*Lentil Salad (315 calories)
5 baby carrots (18 calories)

Total calories = 333

Nicoise Salad

*Nicoise Salad (283 calories)
½ cup strawberries (23 calories)

Total calories = 306

Pan-Fried Chick Peas

*Pan-Fried Chick Peas (313 calories)

Total calories = 313

Peanut Butter & Jelly Sandwich

*Peanut Butter & Jelly Sandwich (284 calories)

Total calories = 284

Peanut Butter Raisin Treat

2 slices light whole wheat bread (140 calories)
1 Tbsp organic peanut butter (105 calories)
25 raisins, layered on sandwich (39 calories)

Total calories = 284

Penne alla Vodka | Papaya

1 cup whole wheat penne (180 calories)
1 cup Vodka sauce from a jar (80 calories)
1 Tbsp Parmigiano-Reggiano cheese, grated (21 calories)
1 cup cubed fresh papaya (27 calories)

Total calories = 308

Penne with Spinach Pesto

*Penne with Spinach Pesto (284 calories)

Total calories = 284

Roasted Tomato Basil Soup | Grilled Cheese

*Roasted Tomato Basil Soup, 1-cup serving (85 calories)
2 slices light whole wheat bread (140 calories)
2 oz fat-free shredded cheddar cheese, melted under broiler (84 calories)

Total calories = 309

Savory Chicken Salad | Raspberries

*Savory Chicken Salad (284 calories)
1 cup raspberries (32 calories)

Total calories = 316

Seared Flank Steak | Cheesy Baked Potato

*1/2 Cheesy Baked Potato (154 calories)
2 ounces thinly sliced flank steak, seared briefly in pan (120 calories)

Total calories = 274

Shrimp Salad | Pita Bread | Grapes

*Shrimp Salad (197 calories)
½ small (4" diameter) whole wheat pita, cut into wedges (37 calories)
20 grapes (68 calories)

Total calories = 302

Steak Salad

*Steak Salad (272 calories)
½ small (4" diameter) whole wheat pita bread (37 calories)

Total calories = 309

Stuffed Pepper | Cantaloupe

*Stuffed Pepper (286 calories)
1 medium wedge of cantaloupe (23 calories)

Total calories = 309

Three-Bean Salad | Turkey Rolls | Grapes

*1/2 serving Three-Bean Salad (153 calories)
4 slices of deli turkey, rolled up (88 calories)
20 seedless grapes (68 calories)

Total calories = 309

Tomato Avocado Salad

*Tomato Avocado Salad (297 calories)

Total calories = 297

TUNA MELT

*Tuna Melt (310 calories)

Total calories = 310

TUNA WRAP

*Tuna Wrap (302 calories)

Total calories = 302

TURKEY AVOCADO WRAP

*Turkey Avocado Wrap (274 calories)
5 baby carrots (18 calories)

Total calories = 290

TURKEY STIR-FRY

*Turkey Stir-Fry (310 calories)

Total calories = 310

VEGGIE PITA

*Veggie Pita (298 calories)
1/2 cup raspberries (32 calories)

Total calories = 330

ZUCCHINI CHICKEN BAKE

*Zucchini Chicken Bake (330 calories)

Total calories = 330

DINNER

*Dinner recipes denoted with an asterisk (*) can be found in 300-Calorie Dinner: 30 Days of Healthy, Hassle-Free Recipes from the editors of Simply Svelte.

BEEF STEW WITH MUSHROOMS

*Beef Stew with Mushrooms (325 calories)

Total calories = 325

BROILED TILAPIA | BROWN RICE | SPINACH WITH LEMON

4-oz tilapia filet, broiled with drizzle of olive oil and thyme (145 calories)
1 cup brown rice (109 calories)
2 cups cooked spinach dressed with lemon and sea salt (41 calories)

Total calories = 295

CHICKEN PICCATA | WILD RICE | ASPARAGUS

*Chicken Piccata, 1 serving (208 calories)
½ cup wild rice (83 calories)
8 spears asparagus (26 calories)

Total calories = 317

Comfort Pasta

*Comfort Pasta (324 calories)

Total calories = 324

Coq au Vin | Mixed Green Salad

*Coq au Vin, 1 serving (235 calories)
2 cups mixed greens with 1 tsp olive oil and 1/2 tsp vinegar (53 calories)

Total calories = 288

Country Fried Steak | Black-Eyed Peas | Collards

*Country Fried Steak, 1 serving (170 calories)
1 cup black-eyed peas, cooked (90 calories)
2 cups collard greens, cooked, seasoned with red pepper flakes (25 calories)

Total calories = 285

CREAMY BEEF GOULASH | MIXED GREEN SALAD

*Creamy Beef Goulash, 1-cup serving (269 calories)
2 cups mixed greens with 1 tsp olive oil and 1/2 tsp vinegar (53 calories)

Total calories = 295

DRUNKEN CHICKEN | BROWN RICE | GREEN BEANS

*Drunken Chicken, one serving (255 calories)
1/4 cup brown rice (55 calories)
1 cup green beans (18 calories)

Total calories = 328

GRILLED CHICKEN | CHEESY RICE | BROCCOLI

Grilled chicken breast, 4-ounce serving (142 calories)
cup brown rice with 1 ounce shredded, melted non-fat cheddar (151 calories)
1 cup raw or lightly steamed broccoli (27 calories)

Total calories = 320

GRILLED SHRIMP | SPAGHETTI ALLA VODKA | CANTALOUPE

8 large grilled shrimp (44 calories)
1 cup whole wheat spaghetti with vodka sauce from a jar (216 calories)
1 Tbsp grated Parmigiano-Reggiano cheese (22 calories)
1 small wedge cantaloupe (19 calories)

Total calories = 301

HAMBURGER | SWEET POTATO

3-oz ground beef patty made with 95% lean beef (139 calories)
1 whole wheat bun (120 calories)
Condiments: 2 romaine leaves, 2 pickles, 1 tsp ketchup, 1 tsp mustard, 1 tomato slice, 1 tsp horseradish (21 calories)
1/2 baked sweet potato with rosemary and sea salt (27 calories)

Total calories = 307

ITALIAN POT ROAST | GREEN BEANS

*Italian Pot Roast, 1 portion (300 calories)
1/2 cup steamed broccoli (30 calories)

Total calories = 330

Lebanese Meatballs | Spinach Salad

*Lebanese Meatballs, 1 serving (264 calories)
2 cups fresh spinach dressed with lemon, oil and vinegar (53 calories)

Total calories = 317

Leg of Lamb | White Beans

4-oz portion of roasted leg of lamb, lean only (203 calories)
1 cup white cannellini beans with rosemary and sea salt (110 calories)

Total calories = 313

Lentil Soup | Spinach Salad

*Lentil Soup (241 calories)
2 cups fresh spinach dressed with lemon, oil and vinegar (53 calories)

Total calories = 294

Mediterranean Mahi-Mahi | Lemon Spinach

6-oz mahi-mahi filet, broiled and topped with 1 tsp olive oil, 1 small chopped tomato, fresh parsley and 5 kalamata olives (266 calories)
2 cups spinach sautéed with lemon and garlic (45 calories)

Total calories = 311

Moroccan Chicken | Flatbread

*Moroccan Chicken, 1 serving (242 calories)
1 small whole wheat flatbread (70 calories)

Total calories = 312

Pan-Fried Pork Chop | Rice | Roasted Cauliflower

1 4-oz boneless pork chop pan-fried with olive oil spray (135 calories)
1 cup brown rice with fresh parsley (109 calories)
2 cups cauliflower roasted in the oven with 1 tsp olive oil (68 calories)

Total calories = 312

PASTA FAGIOLI

*Pasta Fagioli, 1 serving (303 calories)

Total calories = 303

PASTA WITH LEMON AND PARSLEY | GRILLED SHRIMP

*Pasta with Lemon and Parsley, 1 serving (180 calories)
12 large grilled shrimp (65 calories)

Total calories = 292

PENNE WITH MARINARA SAUCE | MIXED VEGETABLES

1 cup (measured dry) whole wheat penne (180 calories)
3 oz marinara sauce from a jar (63 calories)
1 Tbsp grated Parmigiano-Reggiano cheese (22 calories)
1 cup mixed vegetables (40 calories)

Total calories = 305

Pork Chops | Sweet Potato Fries

1 small grilled bone-in pork chop (197 calories)
1 sweet potato, cut into fries, baked with 1 tsp olive oil and rosemary (120 calories)

Total calories = 317

Pork Roast | Root Vegetables | Collard Greens

4-oz serving of pork tenderloin (185 calories)
1 cup roasted root vegetables such as beets, turnips, carrots (75 calories)
2 cups collard greens with red pepper flakes (25 calories)

Total calories = 285

Pork Tenderloin with Apples | Seared Kale

4-oz serving roasted pork tenderloin (185 calories)
1 small apple, roasted (77 calories)
1 cup kale, simmered in water, seasoned with red pepper flakes (34 calories)

Total calories = 296

Salmon Steak | Brown Rice | Broccoli

3-oz serving grilled salmon (175 calories)
1 cup steamed brown rice (109 calories)
1 cup steamed broccoli (31 calories)

Total calories = 315

Southern-Style Minestrone | Mixed Green Salad

*Southern-Style Minestrone, 1-cup serving (240 calories)
2 cups mixed greens with 1 tsp olive oil and ½ tsp vinegar (53 calories)

Total calories = 314

Spaghetti with Clam Sauce

*Spaghetti with Clam Sauce, 1 serving (303 calories)

Total calories = 303

STEAK | ROASTED BEETS | ARUGULA

4-oz lean cut of steak such as sirloin or filet mignon (200 calories)
1 cup fresh beets sliced and roasted with rosemary (56 calories)
2 cups arugula with 1 tsp olive oil and 1 tsp vinegar (53 calories)

Total calories = 305

STUFFED ACORN SQUASH

*Stuffed Acorn Squash (319 calories)

Total calories = 319

TURKEY DINNER | BAKED POTATO | PEAS

4-oz slice of roasted, white meat turkey (158 calories)
1 medium baked potato with 1 pat of fat-free margarine (85 calories)
1 cup cooked green peas (62 calories)

Total calories = 305

VEAL CUTLET DINNER

*Veal Cutlet Dinner (291 calories)

Total calories = 291

Snacks

Avocado | Crackers

1 cup sliced avocado (234 calories)
5 whole wheat crackers (70 calories)

Total calories = 304

Carrots and Sesame Seeds

1 Tbsp sesame seeds (52 calories)
20 baby carrots (70 calories)
1 cup seedless grapes (156 calories)

Total calories = 278

Cheese and Fruit

1 medium pear (96 calories)
3 pieces of light string cheese (180 calories)

Total calories = 276

Cheese and Fruit II

1 cup grapes (104 calories)
5 cubic inches Parmigiano-Reggiano cheese (200 calories)

Total calories = 304

Chips and Salsa

30 plain tortilla chips (264 calories)
3.5 ounces tomato salsa (20 calories)

Total calories = 284

Chocolate and Strawberries

3 cups halved strawberries (146 calories)
2 Tbsp semi-sweet chocolate chips (140 calories)

Total calories = 286

CRACKERS WITH COTTAGE CHEESE

5 rye crackers (97 calories)
4 oz low-fat cottage cheese (100 calories)
1 cup red or green grapes (104 calories)

Total calories = 301

CRACKERS WITH OLIVE SPREAD

5 rye crackers (97 calories)
2 Tbsp black olive tapenade (70 calories)
1 cup red or green grapes (104 calories)

Total calories = 271

DRIED PINEAPPLE RINGS | ALMONDS

2 dried pineapple rings (130 calories)
25 whole almonds (166 calories)

Total calories = 296

Frozen Berries | Yogurt | Almonds

2 cups frozen mixed berries (140 calories)
1 container fat-free Greek yogurt (79 calories)
12 whole almonds (83 calories)

Total calories = 302

Hummus and Veggie Plate

15 baby carrots (53 calories)
20 red pepper strips (5 calories)
20 cucumber slices (17 calories)
1 cup hummus (208 calories)

Total calories = 283

Hummus Sandwich | Raspberries

2 slices whole wheat bread (200 calories)
2 Tbsp hummus (46 calories)
1 cup raspberries (48 calories)

Total calories = 294

MIXED BERRIES | COTTAGE CHEESE | CHEERIOS

1 cup mixed blueberries, raspberries, blackberries (70 calories)
4 ounces low-fat cottage cheese (102 calories)
1 cup dry Multi-Grain Cheerios (110 calories)

Total calories = 282

MIXED NUTS | BLUEBERRIES

1/3 cup mixed nuts (270 calories)
50 blueberries (39 calories)

Total calories = 309

PEANUT BUTTER APPLE | STUFFED GRAPE LEAVES

1 medium apple (77 calories)
1 Tbsp peanut butter (105 calories)
2 dolmades—Greek stuffed grape leaves (134 calories)

Total calories = 316

Peanut Butter Banana | Trail Mix

1 medium banana (105 calories)
1 Tbsp peanut butter (105 calories)
2 Tbsp trail mix (90 calories)

Total calories = 300

Pineapple | Greek Yogurt | Almonds

1 5.3-ounce container of non-fat Greek yogurt (79 calories)
1 cup fresh pineapple chunks (83 calories)
20 whole almonds (139 calories)

Total calories = 301

Popcorn and Peanuts

3 cups popcorn, popped in 2 Tbsp olive or canola oil (165 calories)
20 roasted peanuts (117 calories)

Total calories = 282

Power Smoothie

1 cup fat-free plain yogurt (137 calories), mixed in a blender with:
2 oz fat-free milk (22 calories)
1 cup frozen mixed berries (70 calories)
1 cup chopped fresh mango (54 calories)

Total calories = 283

Pretzels and Cheddar

20 small sourdough pretzels (140 calories)
1 cup cubed cheddar cheese (133 calories)

Total calories = 273

Prosciutto and Melon

3 slices Italian prosciutto ham (210 calories)
20 chunks of cantaloupe or honeydew melon (61 calories)

Total calories = 271

Prosciutto-Wrapped Asparagus

4 slices Italian prosciutto ham, torn in half (280 calories)
8 asparagus spears, boiled and cooled, then wrapped in prosciutto (26 calories)

Total calories = 306

Prosciutto-Wrapped Mozzarella Cheese | Olives

2 slices Italian prosciutto ham (140 calories)
2 oz part-skim mozzarella, wrapped in the prosciutto (144 calories)
3 Nicoise (small black) olives (35 calories)

Total calories = 319

Rice Cereal | Banana

1 cup puffed brown rice cereal (110 calories)
1 cup skim milk (68 calories)
1 medium banana (105 calories)

Total calories = 283

Shrimp Cocktail | Crackers and Cream Cheese

20 large boiled shrimp (109 calories)
2 ounces cocktail sauce (60 calories)
7 whole wheat crackers (105 calories)
1 Tbsp low-fat cream cheese (23 calories)

Total calories = 297

Sunflower Seeds | Grapes

1 cup roasted sunflower seeds (165 calories)
1 cup seedless grapes (156 calories)

Total calories = 321

Tuna Crackers | Olives

5 rye crackers (97 calories)
4 oz water-packed tuna, drained (131 calories)
6 Nicoise (small black) olives (70 calories)

Total calories = 271

Turkey Breadsticks | Cantaloupe

4 sesame breadsticks (200 calories)
4 slices deli turkey, wrapped around the breadsticks (88 calories)
1 small wedge of cantaloupe (20 calories)

Total calories = 308

Veggies with Guacamole

15 baby carrots (53 calories)
20 red pepper strips (5 calories)
4 Tbsp guacamole (200 calories)

Total calories = 258

Yogurt | Pretzels | Strawberries

1 container fat-free, fruit-flavored yogurt (100 calories)
20 small sourdough pretzels (140 calories)
1 cup sliced strawberries (53 calories)

Total calories = 293

ABOUT SIMPLY SVELTE

For years we've been led to believe that exercising is the key to losing weight. The truth is that reaching your ideal weight is 95% eating habits--both the quality and quantity of food that goes in your mouth consistently, each and every day. When you eat clean, track your calories, and make consistent, healthy choices, your weight stays stable--naturally! The Simply Svelte program is not a diet, and is not a fad. It's a sensible way of eating that you'll be able to stick with for life.

Connect with us online at Facebook (Simply Svelte) and Twitter (@SimplySvelte).

OTHER BOOKS BY SIMPLY SVELTE

If you enjoyed this book, check out other recipe and meal planning tools from Simply Svelte. The Simply Svelte team has put together 30 days' worth of healthy, easy-to-prepare breakfasts, lunches, and dinners that will help you lose weight and feel satisfied all day long. With minimal planning, you're on your way to simple, tasty options from Cheese Grits Casserole to Homemade Pizza and Italian Pot Roast. Mix and match the easy, delicious 300-calorie meals in these cookbooks, and you'll be amazed how you look and feel 30 days from today!

Find these books at amazon.com:

300-Calorie Breakfast: 30 Days of Healthy, Hassle-Free Recipes

300-Calorie Lunch: 30 Days of Healthy, Hassle-Free Recipes

300-Calorie Dinner: 30 Days of Healthy, Hassle-Free Recipes

Made in United States
Cleveland, OH
23 January 2025

13716096R00036